Taosool

Taosool

The Art of Standing on One Leg

Chris Milton

ISBN-13: 978-1-7330150-4-2

Published by Backcountry Eagle Productions, Alma, CO.

BackcountryEagle.com

Thank you, Mom and Dad.

Your dedication and hard work are a constant source of inspiration.

Table of Contents

Foreword

In 2008, I began experiencing a migraine that continues daily and the last decade has been spent managing the related issues. The current approach to migraine is short-sighted; we must reevaluate the basic treatment process.

My father and his father before him have suffered from severe migraine, along with a history of this experience on my mother's side that includes prior generations and extends throughout the family tree. I hesitate to even attempt to revisit the past decade, which has been difficult, but my father's recent struggles have inspired me to share my experience.

Until learning about migraines through my personal situation, I knew very little and just thought they were headaches. This is not true, as migraines present in many ways that differ significantly from case to case. A variety of issues have been standardized into a broad category, which leads to vast differences in treatment. Taking ownership of body and mind has been essential for me in controlling migraine.

Through exploration of my migraine management strategies and experiments, I intend to document a unique approach. The baseline symptoms remain, but I have learned to manage the spikes effectively through a series of techniques that can be performed easily without ongoing cost. The journey has been an eye-opening learning experience about the misconceptions involved with migraines. Over time, I deliberately expanded my ability to listen to my core and now my instincts dictate what to ingest and how to exercise my mind and body.

This discussion will begin with considerations around diagnosis and symptoms, before we dive into food, medications, and alternative strategies. My logic is complex not linear; I have attempted to categorize and streamline the topics, although many interrelations must be addressed along the way.

Misdiagnosis

There are significant issues involved with diagnosis and treatment of migraine. The initial steps are focused on medication and waiting to see if other symptoms present. For some, this strategy results in years of indefinite medication. In other cases, this passive approach constitutes a missed opportunity for proactive treatment.

Using hypothetical numbers as an example, assume that one out of every ten thousand people presenting with migraine progresses into a more serious disorder in the short term. The question becomes whether that small chance at proactively identifying a major issue is worth the effort of going through a diagnostic process. Would it be beneficial to run an extra test on ten thousand people if it would save one life? What if the ratio is one in ten? One in a million?

The answer to this question depends on perspective. If cost is the determining factor, the answer is no. On the other hand, many patients will approve a proactive solution, even when it is presented with risks.

I am very glad that I travelled home at a critical time, spending a few weeks with my parents just as things accelerated for my father. Initially the trip was focused on the Red Sox, but they won the series in five games so there was a parade instead of game six. Certainly not a bad outcome, Go Sox! The visit transitioned into migraine support, as my father was in significant pain. Not only was he visibly uncomfortable, but this concern was also taking a toll on my mother.

One consistent factor is that both my father and I appear to have worked through the initial onset of migraine, ignoring the symptoms and finally going to the doctor when we were desperate for relief. This left us highly suggestable during these early visits, willing to accept any potential solutions presented.

The diagnosis of migraine seemed apparent when he went to his primary doctor because of the severe head pain he was experiencing, but also due to the family history. The prescribed treatment was a combination of short-term quick fix medications and long-term medications. When he returned with the initial diagnosis, I provided context from my experience. He was quick to adopt many of the dietary restrictions discussed below, especially the items that were main parts of his diet.

A few weeks later during the consultation with a neurologist, the details around these major steps already taken forced them to consider more complex possibilities. Through this exploration, the specialist uncovered a different major issue. It seems very possible that without the additional confirmation of serious discomfort, the diagnosis would have remained basic.

We will never know how much these few weeks of general treatment impacted the events that followed, but at this point my father's vision is threatened. There is no denying the existence of a period after his misdiagnosis, prior to the start of his correct treatment, that could have been used in a more proactive manner. The right blood test would have shown the true issue earlier. It appears that my father was never suffering from migraine, but he was caught in the net because of the broad nature of this category.

I do not advocate running random tests to eliminate all possibilities, but pharmaceutical roulette to find a treatment that works is not appropriate either. In fact, a course of drugs seems like a more drastic step than a blood test. The decision not to explore further testing is reasonable assuming that there is low risk of complication, but I take issue with the suggestion of medication as an effective first step because it can blur any other potential symptoms with side effects. There are many effective drugs, which I am in favor using when appropriate, but they are not a magic wand. Wouldn't it be better to focus on identification of specific issues, rather than just treatment of a mysterious problem?

To borrow a term from risk management, the current overall medical strategy is avoidance. The first step is to medicate the patient. If that doesn't work and the patient returns, a variety of pharmaceutical categories can be explored, which creates a roadmap for years of drug testing. There seems to be a false assumption that if the medication 'helps' on a self-reported basis, then it is obviously the right treatment. There is apparently no benefit to proactive exploration at the time of initial complaint.

This last part is the key, because if there are minimal serious concerns for a patient presenting with migraine, why treat them at all?

In my case, pharmaceuticals negatively impacted my system, while also making it harder to distinguish the actual symptoms from the side effects. The prescriptions added variables to the equation rather than removing them. I trusted the doctors' confidence in medication as a solution and that ultimately reduced my ability to express my symptoms accurately. I regret that I did not take ownership of my situation earlier. My diagnosis was complicated by the side effects of these medications and the initial treatment delayed my progress.

Medication testing threw me into a pharmaceutical cloud for years. I am optimistic that this phase was abbreviated for my father, but it may have been too long. Would his vision have been saved by an earlier blood test? Are there certain aspects of his symptoms that could have been identified? These are questions that may never be answered.

I recognize the difficulties that doctors face, wading through a sea of issues to find the percentage with major complications. An essential consideration should be to protect against the risk of overmedicating prior to identifying a treatable concern, especially in the context of the current prescription addiction epidemic. My alternate strategy is to focus on migraine management and ongoing monitoring to uncover other symptoms if they present.

Symptoms

My migraine experience started early in my professional career, presenting with a variety of symptoms. At first, I said nothing. Many symptoms are low level and even the spikes are mysterious. Quickly, the issues impacted my ability to focus in a variety of situations. As the concerns escalated, I was forced into action.

Nausea and light sensitivity have been the core of my migraine since the beginning. Other symptoms are involved such as sound sensitivity, pain in a variety of locations, dehydration, disorientation, loss of equilibrium, and even loss of consciousness. This section explores my symptoms while also noting basic management strategies.

Light Sensitivity

This has been the most consistent variable in my decade long migraine and today I try not to venture outside without sunglasses. Direct light, excessive screen time or fluorescent light can exacerbate my symptoms.

The key with light exposure seems to be angle. When direct light from the sun or a lamp enters my eyes, this will certainly lead to a severe migraine spike within seconds to minutes. Often this is accompanied by an aura, where any objects present with a haze around the edges and flashing lights sparkle in the corners of my vision. I also experience an eye twitch, mostly in my left eye. While the twitch seems to be linked to light exposure, it is difficult to draw a direct connection.

The best reaction is to adjust position relative to the light source as quickly as possible. In some cases, there is nothing to be done, while in others it is possible to react and reduce the exposure. When sitting down at a restaurant or other location, I look to see where the light originates and position myself appropriately, preferably with the light on my back rather than in my eyes. At events, this is often harder to control. I have attended a variety of concerts and plays where the stage lights were positioned directly in my eyes, ensuring that I will be riding a migraine spike through the production. When bathed in bright light while my surroundings are dark the onset is accelerated.

In these situations, those around me are usually not bothered by the direct light and I must take control to adjust where possible. If the person across from me is backlit, the aura develops quickly around that figure as I struggle to maintain concentration and eye contact. Especially early in my migraine experience, I would just power through the discomfort, often leaving meetings in a haze with watery eyes. Over time I learned to share my discomfort and react appropriately. Most people are very understanding and a simple request to switch seats or change locations can help, but in some cases that is not possible and other approaches must be developed on the fly.

I refuse to let this hold me back and still spend significant periods outdoors, but it is important to be prepared. When skiing for example, the snow reflects light from the sun, which often triggers discomfort. Instead of not skiing, which to me would be unthinkable, I try to prepare appropriately.

Reducing trigger levels through rest and diet so that my body can handle the load is helpful, but I also carry extra ski goggles in case of an issue with my primary set. During some periods of this journey the migraine has disrupted my favorite activities or foods, but this creates an entirely different type of discomfort. Short term limitations are one thing, but long-term ultimatums are extreme.

That said, the opposite is also true: if you don't enjoy something and it causes your migraine to spike, why would you continue?

Sound Sensitivity

This is an important extension of light sensitivity, but light usually leads the way. Loud noise is less disruptive in a darker context than in a bright situation. This is another trigger that is almost impossible to control so I must accept it and prepare appropriately.

One constant is tinnitus, ringing in the ears, although my hearing is technically strong. Background noise is much more prevalent for me and can take over, causing near field noise to be difficult to isolate. It is challenging to narrow my focus on any single source in loud situations. When I am in a bustling location, carrying on a conversation is difficult.

Taosool can be very effective providing release, as often noise is unavoidable and must be managed. We will discuss this strategy in more detail below, but it is important to note that the mental state attained through Taosool can be accessed in a variety of situations. Meditation has been an effective way to block out noise even when that seems impossible.

Headache

Many would assume that a migraine is a severe headache, but this is a common misconception. This sensation feels as if my head is an overinflated balloon, certainly related to the pressure discussed below. Sometimes mysterious severe pain will present as if a spike were entering my skill at various angles. This is often on the right side of my head, although it migrates throughout my skull muscle structure. In some cases, this pain is focused higher on my skull near my temple or above while in other situations it is closer to my ears, jaw or neck.

Head pain has not been the most disruptive part of my migraine experience, as it tends to be preceded by other symptoms such as light sensitivity and nausea. The other symptoms are more troublesome daily, but during severe spikes headache makes it more difficult to focus on the task at hand.

Pressure

Another area of discomfort is pressure in my sinus cavity. It appears that the Eustachian tube from my sinuses to my inner ear does not function properly. When I am in an environment of changing pressure, it impacts my head very significantly and exacerbates my migraine symptoms.

This is a familiar sensation due to lifelong environmental allergies, experience scuba diving, and a tendency to change elevation frequently. The faster pressure changes, the more it impacts my baseline. There are a series of potential situations, examples include flying in an airplane, driving through a mountain range, or even changing weather pressure. These along with a variety of other triggers cause pressure changes and my head doesn't seem to equalize correctly in response.

The exploration of my ears and sinuses was initiated by me based on my discomfort and the ear specialist quickly identified items that other doctors had ignored. Through hearing testing and physical exams, they isolated the issue with my Eustachian tube. Even though I feel a direct connection between this area and my symptoms, my other doctors refused to draw a correlation, so it remained a separate diagnosis unrelated to migraine. I disagree with this assessment and am confident there is a connection. This lack of response to a related concern underscores the fact that I was required to take ownership of my issues.

The desire by doctors to treat items separately was a frustration I experienced multiple times through this process. At one point, a blood test reflected that my thyroid was not functioning correctly.

The response? More medication.

This new discovery did not cause any change in reaction to the original issue, my doctors just piled another drug on top of the existing prescriptions at the time. Thyroid issues are apparently easily managed through medication, but the mounting list of issues that doctors ignored caused frustration on my end. It felt as if we were making progress isolating concerns, but rather than reevaluating our overall approach when this happened, the new symptoms would be segregated. I am sure this is an appropriate response with some diseases, but with a mysterious diagnosis such as migraine there should be more reaction when new details arise. It is possible that thyroid and/or sinus issues were the true concern from the beginning of my migraine, but my doctors ignored these theories. I spent multiple years overlapping thyroid and migraine medication before ending medication completely.

Planes are a challenge, as the artificial pressurization causes problems for me. I still fly when needed because it is convenient, so I have learned to manage my discomfort. On one severe occasion I was on an airplane and as soon as the door closed, it was as if they flipped a switch in my head and I immediately began to experience motion sickness, although we had yet to pull away from the gate. The symptoms escalated as the plane took off and I vomited repeatedly throughout the flight. Once we made it to our destination and reached the gate, the extreme pressure released, and I recovered quickly.

Using a technique learned in scuba, I equalize when this feeling is extreme, holding my nose and gently forcing air into my sinuses. This can provide relief, but it is essential not to overuse because it can stretch the eardrum. One of my ear doctors along the way described this as pulling on your shirt collar, where a few tugs don't do much and the collar goes back to shape but continued ongoing stretching can cause deformation.

This equalization is a two-step process for me, which is different than many other accounts. Step one is above, where I force air into my sinuses, thus increasing the pressure. The next phase is to swallow, which clears the added pressure and brings me to an equilibrium. This pairs well with neck and head stretches, as these relax muscles and enhance benefit. This strategy can be very effective, sometimes causing an instant release of pressure, but other times it is counterproductive. When not successful, the pressure inside my head increases, but then the return to equilibrium takes time. This type of failure is usually followed by aura, flashing lights in my vision, and escalation of nausea.

Pressure is another variable that is difficult to control, forcing other items to the top of the priority list. When my trigger load is lower overall, I am better prepared to handle changing pressure.

Insomnia

My sleep patterns have varied over time and lack of rest is a significant migraine trigger. With sleep, as with many areas of life, I only worry about what is under my control. It is impossible to force myself to fall asleep; if I get in bed too early, I lay awake indefinitely. Instead of trying to go to sleep at night, I get up early in the morning. The beginning of the day is much easier to manage. By getting up earlier, I am tired earlier, and I fall asleep naturally.

I function best on two sleep cycles, each running two and a half to three hours. Once the third cycle begins it is best to complete it rather than interrupting any cycle in the middle. This is an essential takeaway: I am more rested on less sleep. Natural light is very helpful in managing sleep, waking naturally is healthier than the jolt of an alarm. Exposure to dusk as the light disappears for the day engages our natural instincts.

One step that I explored is a sleep study, which gave me a better understanding of my cycles. This is very beneficial because the sleep lab is detailed in their analysis. The sleep study identified mild central apnea, which means that the signal to breath from my brain to my lungs is mysteriously interrupted periodically. This is different from other types of sleep apnea, which are physiological.

In my case the apnea has never been severe enough to require use of a CPAP machine. Subsequent sleep studies have shown improvement and I intend to repeat the sleep study over time to monitor trends. CPAP stands for Continuous Positive Airway Pressure and the machines create pressure and support breathing by forcing air gently into the airway. Given the sinus pressure considerations above, I am hesitant to introduce CPAP into my routine because it would stress a part of my system that is already struggling to function.

A concern with sleep studies is the built-in problem of sample size. It was easy to settle in for the night and give them sleep data, but that is not representative of a normal night's sleep. Modern technology allows us to monitor this over a longer period and analyze more accurate statistics, rather than only a single night. There are a variety of wearable technologies and bed sensors that can be used, along with most smartphones.

Neck Tension

Much of my pain originates in my neck, although that is a critical area so the discomfort spirals throughout the rest of my body. This is closely linked to sinus pressure and it is unclear which factor drives the other. The upper neck is extremely difficult to release, which has spawned many of my relaxation techniques.

Over time I have worked with a variety of specialists who have different theories on how to reach my target areas. I spent time with masseuses, chiropractors, and even tried acupuncture, all of which contributed to my understanding of basic alignment and realignment.

Massage. A great way to refocus migraine is through massage. I especially found benefit in neck and scalp massage, although the results tended to be short-term. As with many professional areas, there are vast differences between a good and a bad masseuse, but there are also different types and specialties. Comfort is essential, relaxing massage is more beneficial to migraine than deep tissue in my experience.

At one point, I was a member at a massage chain that allowed me flexibility for last minute scheduling in multiple locations. The downside was that most times, I had to repeat my medical and physical history to bring the new provider up to speed. Recounting this information in detail repeatedly caused frustration, especially when all I wanted was a relaxing experience. Sometimes, the masseuse would have insight on customization of a technique, while others would simply go through the motions of a basic massage.

Two masseuses are worthy of consideration, one through this chain and another outside of that system. The specific masseuse at the chain was a young mother who had also struggled with migraine for years and she was able to target areas more accurately based on my commentary. It was clear that her empathy for this mysterious issue assisted her ability to provide unique solutions, although our schedules did not align so the sessions were limited in number.

The other masseuse was outside this system and had much more experience treating a variety of issues through the years. She was a referral from a good friend, which created a level of immediate trust. I provided background on my issues, but she was able to sense my areas of discomfort without any direction. Especially in subsequent sessions, there was little need to discuss details. On multiple occasions she encouraged engagement of other specialists where needed.

One such specialist was a chiropractor, who worked together with her to release my target areas. On another occasion, she correctly identified the need for a foot and ankle specialist during my recovery from a torn Achilles. The long-time experience of this independent masseuse made a significant difference.

Chiropractor. Much of my pain is focused at the top of my spine where it connects to my skull, which is a very difficult area to target. Early in my migraine experience I tested a few introductory sessions with a chiropractor who taught me basics. Early in my life, I cracked my knuckles and various other joints like my neck. This is not a good habit and I have limited it over time, but the long-term impact remains. Due to this history, the chiropractor reminded me of that sensation and created an element of hesitation for me.

My trusted masseuse convinced me to explore this option again. It was clear to her that the upper vertebra of my neck was locked into my lower skull and there was limited independent movement. We did a series of combined therapies where she would massage the target area to relax the muscles prior to the neck realignment, along with the reverse where the chiropractor would perform an alignment before massage so that the muscles could be relaxed in line with the adjustment.

While these sessions were beneficial, ongoing visits were required for relief. The treatment was very helpful unlocking areas and gaining an understanding of my body, but long-term it is better to attain this alignment naturally.

Acupuncture. Another type of specialist that I visited along my journey was an acupuncturist. I heard many positive reviews of acupuncture and so I tried it and gave the provider an idea of my migraine history at that point. The sessions were incredibly powerful, requiring significant focus and meditation. The release I felt afterward was undeniable, possibly due to the high intensity of the sessions.

The results were short-lived, and I would usually experience a rebound spike within hours. I discontinued after a few sessions, but I do not discourage anyone from exploration. After this attempt to incorporate acupuncture, I have discussed this topic with others who are involved in the field. While the provider I worked with seemed to have appropriate credentials, this is clearly an area where the right specialist makes a difference.

Time. I often joked that the best thing about massage was that it forced me to lay down and close my eyes for an hour in the middle of the day. Rather than making my body relax through use of a professional in any of these categories, I dedicate that time to Taosool. The hour is much more productive for both body and spirit without having to change locations. I do not currently see any specialists regularly, although I still use a sensory deprivation tank to enhance my meditation and relaxation skills. More detail on floating is below, but time dedicated to Taosool is more beneficial than sessions with any of these specialists.

Disorientation

This is difficult to describe, as it is surreal. While this word can be used in multiple contexts, I intend a direct interpretation because my perception of orientation within my environment changes. Usually disorientation occurs when I am already experiencing the other symptoms and then at a certain moment my environment shifts. It is as if I were turning my head to one side or the other, although I am not moving. This is usually accompanied by a mysterious release of energy, which manifests visually and audibly.

When this occurs, sitting is helpful if available, but I usually try to find a handhold when standing to ensure I have a third point of contact if disorientation worsens. This sensation only lasts a few seconds to a few minutes and often leads to a rapid improvement in symptoms after the episode. I theorize that this is linked to sinus pressure, whereby extreme pressure release causes the experience described above.

On one occasion, I lost consciousness while sitting at my desk at work. I remember trying to continue working even as I could barely focus on my screen, I was determined to push through a severe migraine spike. I woke up on the floor with my team around me. They had already called 9-1-1 and I was transported to the hospital. Mind you, this was not at the beginning of the issue, as I had been experiencing symptoms for an extended time already and this day was explained away by doctors as a system overload. The doctors downplayed this incident, which has always perplexed me. It has never happened since, although it was a catalyst for the extreme dietary measures and other changes to my routine that continue through today.

Nausea

This belongs at the top of the list next to light if these were ordered in terms of consistency, nausea is another symptom that is constant, although it ebbs and flows in severity.

I have experienced motion sickness for my entire life, but early in life it presented in classic motion scenarios such as on boats and in cars or airplanes. Now, I am always motion sick regardless of location. This isn't a perfect analogy, but it is as if I am always on the verge of getting sick (even though I rarely vomit due to migraine).

Diet has a significantly positive impact in this area, but that has not always been easy because nausea can take away the appeal of food. During the worst periods, all my food tasted like ash, which removed my desire to eat. This impact on my taste buds may have been a side effect of medication, as it has improved over time even while the nausea has remained. Regardless of cause, for an extended time there was no joy or satisfaction in any meal because of this issue. I ate only to maintain nutrition.

I theorize that the removal of medication contributed to the improvement, but I am confident that focus on diet also helped regain my love of food. Through the process of discovery described below, I was able to identify items that exhibited both positive and negative impacts on my system. I have continued to adjust the details over time, targeting various foods that are beneficial while limiting anything else.

Drinking small amounts of water consistently helps me manage the nausea. Often, I will take water into my mouth and allow it to soak in slowly. This is a very effective strategy because it is possible to ingest too much water, so allowing it to settle in my mouth extends the benefit of drinking water while minimizing the risk of overhydration. On most days, I drink close to a gallon of still water, a practice that began early in the process when I was experimenting with a variety of prescription medications. One of the side effects of the medication was dehydration, but even in the absence of prescriptions there is a significant positive impact from appropriate hydration. Altitude is worth noting in this context, as I spend significant periods of time over ten thousand feet in a dry environment, which obviously increases hydration requirements.

I enjoy sparkling water immensely; it allows me to continue hydrating while adding variety. I treat myself with soda, but most soda cravings are satisfied with sparkling water. It is easy to add simple juices or natural flavors (pomegranate, agave nectar), but plain sparkling water is my preference. Many confuse this with tonic water or club soda, but these are very different because of sodium content.

Ginger is a one of my favorite foods and it has natural properties that calm the stomach. My mother deserves credit here, this was one item included in my diet since childhood. There are many ways of introducing this into a diet; but ginger ale and fresh ginger are the most effective. Powdered ginger does not seem have as much impact. Fish and sushi are considered below, but the pickled ginger that accompanies sushi is my favorite way to include this in my diet.

This variety of issues has combined to disrupt my system for over a decade. The key takeaway here is the mysterious nature of the symptom's timing and severity. I believe that this is due to the long list of constantly changing variables at any given time. Because of inconsistencies involved with the symptoms described, a flexible strategy is necessary to minimize impact on daily life.

Social Impact

The social impact of migraine is difficult for me to document because I am obviously biased. A few years into this experience, I self-imposed isolation. Explaining my issues and dietary restrictions was tiresome and repetitive. It is much easier to avoid situations where my triggers are present, rather than confronting them directly. I try not to make my migraine a constant topic of discussion, so it is difficult to navigate these situations even now. Shared meals, public events, and backcountry expeditions all present challenges.

In elementary school my friend often had to leave class or events due to migraine. I did not understand what she was going through and certainly did not express empathy for her mysterious issues. Coming full circle, a different friend directly questioned the validity of my symptoms during the early onset of migraine, adding to my insecurity. I respect the fact that my friend expressed his opinion, I am confident that others shared his concerns and were not willing or able to discuss them. I still question whether my initial doctor ever believed my concerns.

I deliberately reversed this isolation trend in recent years, but there are still many situations that must be managed in order to minimize impact. I struggle to maintain eye contact in bright locations, and it is challenging to carry on a conversation in loud areas. These issues result in a lack of social connection during many scenarios. There are times where I can feel that my discomfort is apparent, but I believe this is often misinterpreted by others as lack of interest in the person or the discussion. The only solution for these concerns is to attack them directly by sharing details rather than ignoring them. This is easier said than done because whenever I bring up my migraine in public, it feels like I am complaining. Most people are understanding and many share similar concerns personally and through their family or friends.

During the initial onset, I was still proving myself in the workforce. This made it difficult for me to show weakness. I grew concerned that an error would arise because I was functioning below full capacity, and this led me to take time away from work to regain my abilities. This is a feeling that compares to my recovery from knee surgery, which contained a period where my knee was technically strong, but I still had a mental block about trusting the knee. From what I understand, this is a common phenomenon involved with injury rehab in general. Over time, as I pushed the limits of my abilities, my confidence in that knee returned and now I trust it more than ever.

Similarly, I reached a point after the loss of consciousness where I was out of work for weeks. I had very low confidence in my ability to avoid errors in a fast-paced trading environment. This period away from work forced me to face the decision of allowing the migraine to dominate my life or conquering it and moving forward. Giving in to the migraine is an unacceptable choice, so I returned to work motivated to overcome.

Quick Fixes

A major change arrived during the recovery from my loss of consciousness incident, when I stopped looking for the quick fix solution and accepted the symptoms as my personal reality. The assumption that there is a magical migraine fix is misleading (for me, at least). Our society is focused on instant gratification and everyone from patients to doctors can fall into this trap. Many of the various options could help along the way, but also can create issues of their own.

Eliminating quick fixes is discussed in "How to Heal your Headache: The 1-2-3 Program for Taking Charge of your Pain"[1], by Dr. David Buchholz. In chapter three, encompassing step one, he goes into detail about the various categories of quick fixes and the reasons for and against, including information that is much better provided by a doctor. I was long past any use of quick fix drugs by the time I read The 1-2-3

Program[1], but there is a compelling case including a comprehensive discussion of specific drugs and the rebound effect.

While in my situation it was beneficial to eliminate pharmaceuticals, another case may have different characteristics. Additionally, some find various categories of pharmaceuticals to be helpful. I have intentionally separated this initial discussion of quick fixes from the discussion below about pharmaceutical quick fixes. This is to emphasize my belief that a quick fix could be anything. A cup of coffee, a glass of wine, a yoga pose, a certain comfort food, or anything else that could be introduced during discomfort to improve the situation.

Dr. Buchholz eludes to the distinction, but his consideration of these quick fixes is very focused on drugs that cause rebound. In my view, the essential component to this step does not require stopping or starting any specific strategy, it is about mental expectations. Treatment should be considered in a longer-term light, which can help the broader trends of migraine emerge. Reducing migraine on a single day may be an essential short-term goal, but instant gratification strategies could be detrimental to long term success[1] (Buchholz, Loc 730-1041).

Food

While there are many potential triggers, food is one of the easiest to control. This is certainly a lesson I learned from chapter 4 of The 1-2-3 Program[1], which explores reducing triggers and was the catalyst for my dietary changes (Buchholz, Loc 1046-1742). I can now attest to the power of controlling diet, as my daily strategy revolves around this variable. Through the testing process, I expanded my relationship with food by learning about what I eat and where it is sourced. I prioritize the positives and negatives of each option, balancing these considerations. I eat what I like and consume reasonable amounts spread throughout the course of the day. By trusting myself and listening to my system, I sense what my body craves and rejects.

There are many foods that I have added and subtracted from my diet, but it is essential to take these examples with a grain of salt. Do not assume that anything I tested would provide the same result in another case. I believe that the testing itself is beneficial and has contributed to my knowledge and enjoyment of food. This testing should be approached as a positive factor, an opportunity to explore the world of food, rather than a requirement to eliminate certain items.

My dietary changes were born out of necessity. I was struggling to function daily, working my way along in a pharmaceutical fog. I was desperate and would have tried anything. When I began taking steps to control my diet, I was very strict about certain areas and removed everything that I felt could be contributing to my migraine issues. This included around four years of elimination diet that included caffeine, chocolate, processed meats and foods, alcohol, cheese, citrus, nuts, MSG, fresh bread, and a handful of other items, many of which were included in The 1-2-3 Program[1] (Buchholz, Loc 1205-1472). I prefer to stay positive and will discuss what I have been able to enjoy while also considering the items I limited. I began this extreme step with a static list, but over time my personal list changed through testing.

By simplifying my diet, I now feel the impact of everything I put into my system with much more accuracy. Using this sensitivity, I target things that make me feel good while continuing to limit anything that seems to exacerbate my issues. I say limit, *not eliminate*, because it is more effective to be realistic about expectations. I am confident that there is a 'quality of life' variable that must be considered and depriving myself of favorite foods indefinitely is cruel and unusual punishment.

I generally try to eat fresh and natural foods. While this has required practice, it is a very enjoyable way to eat. I focus on meat at the core of my diet supplemented by a variety of fruits, vegetables, seeds, grains, and snacks. At no point have I felt the need to eliminate any specific spices, which allows me to vary flavor of meats and dishes without having to resort to chemicals.

I treat myself with many triggers in small quantities, which has worked as a reward system and expanded my appreciation for these foods. By remaining disciplined for periods of time, I can take advantage of opportunities when they are presented in the normal course of life.

One of the essential things about my diet is the flexible nature. I try to eat smaller amounts more frequently when my body dictates. This helps keep my energy level consistent while avoiding the food coma caused by large meals. Another important consideration is also dehydration; often when I feel hungry it is thirst for water.

Testing

How do I test these items?

Initially, an important step in my process was eliminating dietary triggers[1] (Buchholz, Loc 1205-1210). I accomplished this through extreme dietary restrictions for approximately four years. As that time passed, I became more in tune with what I put in my system and how it affected me. If I remained strict, how would I ever find out what foods caused a reaction?

Rather than rocking the boat too significantly, I wait for appropriate times to explore each potential trigger. I am a statistician by nature, so I attempt to increase the sample size of the study while isolating variables. This is an ongoing process and I must remain diligent in many areas. The key to an accurate overall evaluation is trying the exact same item in many different situations. By testing under changing conditions, I expand my personal trigger study over time. My intent is grounded in the massive number of variables, although I recognize that this is not strict scientific method.

Flexibility is key, rather than locking into assumptions. It is difficult to remain impartial in my evaluation, so I continuously question results.

This process is incredibly beneficial to both body and mind. Sometimes test results are validating, while in other situations the outcome is unexpected, causing me to reconsider the impact of that trigger along with any other variables that may have been in play.

When I am already having difficulties, there is significant trigger impact. For instance: if exhausted after a poor night's sleep or long day of work, then I am more exposed to a migraine reaction from any trigger. In contrast, I can allow myself leeway with less impact after a period with consistency of diet, sleep, stress, and any other applicable variables. Clearly, the baseline trigger load is very important to consider in any test.

The extreme approach to baseline may have helped my ability to feel the impact of these various items, but I am unsure whether that step is required within the process. Limiting exposure to various categories could reduce trigger loads over time without the need for an elimination diet. The concern with a vague approach is that depending on what is chosen, it could either shorten or extended the process. One possible outcome is that early items being removed from the diet are significant triggers, which could lead to early success, but if the wrong items are isolated first it could lead to discouragement. Even in the first scenario where early results are good, without ongoing evaluation it would be easy to miss other major triggers or slide back into the old patterns.

I continue to test everything and focus on foods with lower impact. I use more of the acceptable foods while experimenting with different additions. Instead of diving further into statistical theory around sample sizes, it seems much more helpful to consider specific examples from my experience.

Spices

Starting with spices is appropriate because it is a category that can be combined with every other food in order to add variety. As I explored the food groups, this is one broad category that did not cause any apparent issues for me.

My favorite spices include rosemary, thyme, sage, basil, oregano, cilantro, and many different peppers (discussed in more detail below). Certain flavors do not agree with me, such as garlic and onions, but this is more of a preference than a migraine decision. Since these two are very common, I must be creative to avoid them.

There is a big difference between actual spices and rubs or spice medleys. Many of the pre-packaged combinations include additives that can be triggers, but they can also contain undesired flavors such as garlic. In the beginning I spent energy reading labels and trying to identify which were acceptable, but it is much easier to simplify this approach and focus in on the fundamental spices. This is like exploring the spectrum of colors, where there are only a few primary colors, but by mixing them in different concentrations a broad variety emerges. The flavor of core foods is easily manipulated through combinations of spices[1] (Buchholz, Loc 1399-1405).

The exploration of spices has been an enjoyable part of this food journey. Pasta is one dish that can be changed significantly using spices. Shapes and sizes of noodle can also be adjusted to add variety. While I often use a tomato or alfredo sauce, my favorite is to add butter or olive oil and spices without additional sauce, which allows for vast differences in flavor while maintaining simplicity. Many noodles contain gluten, which is another trigger discussed below.

Fruits and Vegetables

Fruits and vegetables are generally categorized for the purposes of this discussion, but there are many subsets that should be considered. This area includes a variety of foods that do not impact my migraine. For my entire life I have been a carnivore, eating mostly meat and avoiding many veggies. My limited diet leading into the elimination period created added challenges implementing restrictions and forced me to expand my vegetable horizons. I am still a novice, but the exploration has been enjoyable and successful.

Lettuce is bland, but it can be tolerated. I prefer kale or spinach greens, both of which can be used as a natural base for smoothies. Potatoes are a foundational food; there are many different varieties that can easily be roasted with brussel sprouts, olive oil, and spices. Broccoli and cauliflower would only have been eaten out of necessity and are now staples of my diet, they can be steamed or added to the veggie roast above.

Onions and garlic have never agreed with my system and when I have tried to introduce them it has not been successful; some have reported issues here while others continue to enjoy them. This is a perfect example of the personal exploration I have discussed, as it is important to determine the actual impact of each area rather than the assumed impact.

Buchholz[1] correctly identified bananas as an issue for me (Loc 1417-1420, 1444-1452). I avoid these completely and am very careful not to make a mistake. Prior to the restrictions, banana bread or just simple bananas were a staple breakfast for me, but I have adjusted. Attempts to test or reintroduce have resulted in both short-term impact and long-term baseline shift.

Peppers. All types of peppers[1] are acceptable to me (Buchholz, Loc 1399-1405). I am a fanatic for everything from hot to sweet peppers, these are a great way to supplement and vary flavor of core dishes. I enjoy experimenting with hot peppers and through exploration of the extremes my ability to taste the entire spectrum of peppers has improved. Relatively common and easy to access are Habanero and Bhut Jolokia (Ghost Pepper).

Habanero is certainly hot when used in high concentrations, but it is very sweet in the correct proportions. The other thing worth noting about habanero is the differences between parts of the pepper, as the seeds and upper flesh contain most of the spice and the tip of the pepper is often relatively sweet. This will vary from pepper to pepper so managing the amount of spice can be difficult, dried peppers last longer and are often easier to cook with when ground.

Ghost Peppers are incredibly hot, at one time the hottest measured pepper on earth, but they are worth exploring. An interesting aspect is that they do not add much flavor to a dish on the front end, mostly arriving during the aftertaste. As a result, pairing cayenne and black pepper with ghost pepper increases the front-end spice while still allowing the ghost to dominate the back end.

The spice in this pepper builds so it is essential to avoid over spicing any dish. The first bite will rarely result in a reaction, but after multiple bites the spice will intensify. Ghost pepper is much easier to handle when ground, it is useful as steak rub or to sprinkle into pasta sauce. I learned the hard way what it feels like to inhale and contaminate eyes; caution is recommended when handling any hot pepper, gloves and mask are helpful.

These peppers can expand the flavor of many foods when used in appropriate amounts, but overuse should be avoided. Consumption of hot peppers creates an adrenaline response, which may vary the balance of migraine, but it is a potential quick fix trap. A recent example of using hot peppers to directly control my migraine was on a long flight, which can make me very uncomfortable as discussed. In this case, I was incredibly successful combating the issues involved with an extended flight. There was a surprisingly good meal served, including a curry that came with a hot pepper. Rather than mix in the pepper, I slowly enjoyed the relatively mild curry, along with the rest of the provided meal. After dinner, I cut the pepper into pieces, consuming small amounts at a time along with large amounts of water. I was still in a state of pressure discomfort, but both the food and the hot pepper provided an ongoing distraction.

This is a good example of my strategy personalization on the fly, where I introduced positive elements in a careful way to balance the negativity of my migraine. We will discuss Taosool in detail later, but it is worth noting that I also spent significant amounts of time on this extended flight performing the base motions of Taosool in the galley of the plane.

Citrus. I am impacted by all citrus[1] (Buchholz, Loc 1413-1417). The acidic content contributes to nausea, but in small amounts I can tolerate it. This allows for inclusion as a garnish or minor component, while still limiting most citrus juices and sodas containing high levels of citric acid.

This limitation raises obvious concerns around lack of vitamin C, so I have been careful to add this back into my diet in other ways. Red bell peppers are a wonderful source of vitamin C, they have become one of my favorite snacks and I eat them by hand just as many eat apples. I am sure there are similar issues with exposure or lack of exposure to other nutrients due to my unique diet; any restrictions or additions must be considered in a broad nutritional context.

Berries. Always a favorite of my family, I am especially drawn to strawberries, blueberries, and raspberries. I encountered grey area in this category as well, with raspberries causing short term escalation of nausea, but strawberries and blueberries are acceptable[1] (Buchholz, Loc 1414).

Raspberries have evolved into one of the hardest triggers to avoid so I treat myself when I feel the time is right. Since I have clearly identified them as a trigger, there is minimal testing required. I wait until a time when I am at a good baseline level and raspberries are available in the normal course of life. At that point, I will take advantage of them while trying to moderate intake.

A favorite desert is chocolate cake with raspberries. The chocolate is also a potential trigger so it can be substituted for vanilla ice cream or other deserts as discussed below. Raspberries are also an excellent topping for oatmeal, pancakes, and waffles for breakfast, but other berries can be easily substituted. Strawberries and blueberries can be added to a variety of breakfast and desert dishes to add flavor and color.

Meat

Many have eliminated this category completely for a variety of reasons, resulting in vegetarian, vegan, or pescatarian diets. I encourage personal exploration and provide this detail on my choices for context, but I do not look to force my diet on anyone. While I am certainly a carnivore, these choices could easily be adapted to the individual. The underlying theory of testing and trigger isolation is the focus, rather than the specific foods I have chosen over time.

There are a variety of meats, so distinction must be made; I have separated fish below and intend to discuss land-based meat under this heading. This broad category can be separated further, and I generally think of all deli meats and aged meats such as jerky to be processed meat. While all meat can develop migraine trigger chemicals, the processed meats are a more likely culprit[1] (Buchholz, Loc 1359-1368).

Classifications of nitrate free deli meats are misleading because any curing process naturally creates similar chemicals. My tests of any difference in these deli meats have been inconclusive and so I remain strict, removing them from my normal cycle and only resorting to use when there are no alternatives. Regardless of cured vs uncured or nitrate free vs standard deli, most packaged meats impact my system in a negative way. Processed meats cause a baseline shift, where small amounts are unnoticeable, but multiple consecutive days of intake adds up to a problem. To avoid this implication, I focus on fresh or frozen cuts of actual meat. One example of a difference is turkey, where fresh turkey is acceptable, but deli turkey impacts me significantly.

I have successfully reintroduced some processed meats, but I remain strict on deli meats. This is an easier category to avoid completely rather than parsing the differences in good deli meat and bad deli meat. Jerky is a very beneficial snack and while I have added it back to my trail food, I still limit when possible. One expedition where my jerky intake was high seemed to impact my baseline, so I remain careful with this category, but the variety of jerky makes it very convenient in the backcountry (elk, buffalo, beef, turkey, bacon, etc.).

To increase variety of meat while limiting processed meat, I expanded my repertoire of cuts. It is easy to ensure that the core choices do not become tiresome by shifting between more marbled cuts and lean meats.

My favorite cut of beef is by far the ribeye, due to the variety of fat content in a single cut. Very little preparation is required, although it takes practice to cook a ribeye properly. I tend to use a simple pepper and spice rub, then cook through on one side until the meat is sweating visibly before flipping. I have found that if you don't cook through on this first flip, it is extremely difficult to finish correctly. The ribeye can be contrasted with tenderloin, sirloin, and strip steak cuts for classic steaks or other cuts such as roasts or flank steak to add variety. Ground beef can easily be utilized for burgers, pasta sauce, or tacos. Selection is essential, it is important to source this meat in the best way possible, preferably in a sustainable manner.

Buffalo is an excellent addition because it tends to be leaner than beef and is available in similar cuts. Lamb is another useful red meat, chops are the most common, but shanks and steaks are wonderful. Depending on location there are many others to be explored, such as elk, duck, or venison.

Pork is a staple that can be used in a variety of dishes. Tenderloin and chops can be grilled or broiled; both absorb flavor incredibly well. Bacon is a difficult tradeoff, as it is generally cured and certainly causes a reaction, but for me it is worth eating in moderation because it is incredibly good with eggs and other staples. Even some potential alternatives such as turkey bacon have impact, which is why I have returned to classic bacon rather than using a replacement. With bacon specifically, the main processed meat that I have reintroduced, I buy slabs of unflavored bacon and cut it into pieces before freezing in small portions for easier preparation. Here again is an example of managing the issue to allow enjoyment of favorites; I accept limited exposure to bacon, but I restrict additives.

Chicken is another option that absorbs various flavors. There are vast differences between fresh chicken and the frozen options. Beware of chicken fingers and chicken nuggets as they tend to be covered in MSG[1] (Buchholz, Loc 1313-1359). You can make your own tenders if needed by breading and frying strips of chicken breast, but I tend to limit the gluten in this area and focus on whole chickens, breasts, wings, or thighs.

Many different cuts of chicken can be prepared easily. It is simple and consistent to bake chicken in an oven. The time varies depending on what part is in use, but an hour at four hundred degrees is a general rule of thumb if I am baking large chicken breasts with no bones. Trial and error are required here because conditions such as altitude will impact cooking times. Most meats come out more tender when cooked long and low, but this is a balancing act with available time. Meat thermometers can be helpful if unsure of cook times, but there is no replacement for practice.

By rubbing dry or fresh spices onto the meat, it is easy to infuse interesting flavors and vary a dish. This can be contrasted with use of a wet sauce or marinade, many of which have a vinegar base, another potential trigger that must be tested[1] (Buchholz, Loc 1393-1398).

Again, I recognize that not everyone chooses to include meat in their diet, and I encourage personal choices. Whether or not you eat meat, this exploration process should be focused on whatever foods you enjoy. The key takeaways here are variety and customization, regardless of category it is essential to test each individual component.

Fish

I consider this meat, but since it has unique characteristics it is worthy of separate consideration. Just as with other types, distinction must be drawn between fresh and processed. Smoked and aged meats cause reactions while fresh fish is a very clean meal. Raw fish is enjoyable if high quality, but many cooked fish are also excellent[1] (Buchholz, Loc 1359-1368).

Cooked shrimp, lobster and crab are useful additions for variety because they contrast with other food. Ocean fish such as swordfish and river fish such as salmon or trout add textures and flavors.

Sushi is one of my favorite meals, but it tends to carry a hefty price tag. Sushi grade fish is available at good fish markets and allows for larger portions without escalating cost. Simple choices such as tuna are best for home preparation, as other varieties can require more specific training. Even in restaurants, I lean toward the more simplistic options of nigiri sushi (sliced fish on rice) and sashimi (fish with no rice), rather than complex rolls. I still enjoy some sushi rolls, but I am careful to identify any potential triggers during the ordering process. Creative rolls using soy paper and cucumber rather than traditional seaweed can also add variety. The ginger mentioned earlier may contribute to the lack of nausea caused by this meal, but I also find the spice of wasabi to be enjoyable. Traditional soy sauce contains gluten, there are gluten free options available, but I prefer the real thing in moderation.

Rice

Many of the foods discussed already can be combined well with rice. This is highly effective in adding volume and flavor variety. Some consider this one item, but it is a broad category and there are different types of rice to be explored. Spices can be very useful when pairing rice with other parts of a meal and I prefer adding these spices during cooking to infuse flavor. I also add butter to my rice, which increases flavor and fat content. Many will argue here that fat is bad, but in moderation it is very beneficial, especially in the backcountry.

Nuts

Nuts have been a personal exploration, as some of my favorites (pecans, walnuts, peanuts) cause immediate chalkiness in my throat and trigger nausea over time, forcing me to remain strict. Many other nuts have not caused any reaction (pistachios, almonds, cashews). During times of strict adherence, when all nuts were off limits, I replaced the nutty sensation with seeds, oats, and non-nutty granola.

My father is the master of pecan pie, which has made this result very difficult for me. I have tested pecans repeatedly under many different conditions and in every case the chalky taste arrives quickly. There have been many examples of triggers that I have successfully reintroduced, but this is one category where I must remain diligent. Customization is critical because I do not expect this list of nut issues (or other foods) to be the same for everyone[1] (Buchholz, Loc 1391-1393).

Dairy

Most dairy is acceptable to me, with the main exception of cheese. I use milk sparingly as an addition to coffee or eggs, but it is not a trigger for me. When nausea is extreme milk can help calm the stomach short term, although any benefit to nausea is short lived.

Cheese[1] is a perfect example of ongoing discipline paired with flexibility (Buchholz, Loc 1368-1390). I feel the impact of many cheeses on my system, but still enjoy occasional treats. Generally, the impact is both short and long term as they disrupt digestion, cause mild nausea, and impact my baseline for days to weeks. Instead of never eating cheese, I have eliminated it from my normal rotation. When I encounter an incredible cheese, I allow myself to enjoy it without guilt.

While processed cheeses do not cause the same reaction, I found it easier to eliminate all cheese rather than tempt myself with inferior cheese. This also simplifies restaurant issues because what kind of cheese they use is no longer relevant.

Bread

I have felt impact from gluten, but rather than eliminate it completely I try to manage my intake. Here again there is family history, but testing has shown that I am gluten intolerant and I have not presented with celiac disease.

Fresh breads[1] (Buchholz, Loc 1428-1434) are a more significant trigger for me than packaged bread, but these same fresh breads are my preference. Just as with cheese, I prefer to avoid all breads rather than incorporate less enjoyable varieties. I have limited most bread on a consistent basis in order to allow for flexibility when needed, thus I am able to enjoy special breads on occasion.

To accomplish this, I have removed basic items such as sandwiches that use bread. Throughout my life, peanut butter and honey (a twist on the classic PB+Jelly) was a staple lunch or snack, but since the bread and peanuts both impact me I have removed this favorite from the rotation. I still often find myself in a situation where breaded food is the only option, at which point I decide if a small amount is reasonable or if I should remain strict.

Another longtime favorite is ham on a roll. Many prefer complex sandwiches loaded with a variety of options, but I have always enjoyed a simple sub roll loaded with ham. I ran five-thousand-meter (5K) cross country in high school and this was my pre-race food, adding to the sentimental attachment. Both ham and the roll are triggers so I have eliminated this as a standard choice, although I still visit my hometown deli for occasional nostalgia.

One of the main breads that I use to treat myself is hamburger or hot dog buns. Here, I use a hybrid strategy to reduce intake while enjoying the classic style. The first few bites including the bun maintains the traditional flavor combination. When appropriate, I remove the remaining bread and finish the meat separately. Hot dogs are also in the category of processed meats discussed above and can contain significant amounts of nitrates, but I have been enjoying franks at the ballpark for my entire life, so I still partake.

Pepperoni pizza is another favorite for as long as I can remember, but it is the migraine triple threat. Bread, processed meat, and cheese[1] (Buchholz, Loc 1428-1434, 1368-1390, 1360-1368). While I was strict for a time, I now use it as a treat. Because I avoid these items in most situations, pizza is an option when appropriate.

A potential overlap with bread is beer, also a source of significant gluten. We will discuss alcohol in general below, but since I have reintroduced both beer and bread in moderation it is critical not to overlap. If I am enjoying a beer, I try not to add bread to the equation, and vice versa. Combining triggers is not generally a good idea, but certain items overlap more than others. The extreme overlap in this case seems to indicate gluten as the underlying trigger.

Deserts

Chocolate was the most difficult to limit at first because of my sweet tooth. Other foods are much harder to avoid long term. I have now successfully reintroduced chocolate in moderation, but more than a small amount leads to nausea and dehydration. Real chocolate contains caffeine as well, which is another major trigger[1] (Buchholz, Loc 1260-1313).

Sweets are a reward system in my diet, a strategy my parents taught me early that has continued into my strict dietary pattern. Creativity was required in exploring items that did not include chocolate. Ice cream and its various cousins (sorbet, shaved ice, etc.) filled a large part of this void. Sugar candy of many types including jelly beans can be another replacement for chocolate, but these carry their own health concerns and must be managed appropriately.

Pie and cake are acceptable, depending on ingredients. Many flavors are available, but a few of my favorites are pumpkin, apple, and blueberry. In either case, scratch ingredients tend to be better than store bought cake filled with preservatives. Often the crust will contain gluten, which must be considered.

Maple sugar is a great replacement because the sugar candy tends to contain less additives and pure syrup can be used on many different items. I prefer waffles and pancakes, which are often considered breakfast, but can make a wonderful meal at any time of day!

As with other categories, there is similarity in trigger load to consider. Chocolate contains caffeine so adding this to coffee or soda can duplicate exposure. Another compound impact in this category is sugar and alcohol, which is a common combination. Essentially any desert combined with alcohol will overlap, which often requires creativity or moderation.

This is another highly personalized area that must be tested, I am strict without sacrificing quality of life. By remaining disciplined at certain times, I successfully reward myself with favorites when appropriate.

Caffeine

My relationship with caffeine has evolved over the years, so context seems necessary. I grew up mostly without coffee, since both my parents are tea drinkers. Soda was the main caffeine involved in my early life, although it was limited at home. Sunkist remains a longtime favorite that I use as a reward.

When I was in college, my espresso habit took hold. What at first began with shots of espresso eventually turned to cups of espresso and by the time I entered the workforce it was entrenched in my routine. My work was intense and required long hours, which only compounded the caffeine addiction. Coffee was always available in the office and I progressed into significant energy drink consumption. This period of excessive caffeine may have been a contributing factor to the initial development of my migraine, although high stress and lack of sleep were also at extremes during this period.

As I implemented restrictions, caffeine was one that I knew to be an obvious culprit and so I was strict in the elimination period. This removed coffee and energy drinks from my diet, but also required discipline involving chocolate and soda, along with anything that contained trace amounts of caffeine. Herbal tea was a wonderful replacement, but there is a difference between anything with 'no caffeine' as compared to 'decaffeinated'. Most green or black teas contain caffeine, which means that the herbal teas must be simple and generally fruit or berry based[1] (Buchholz, Loc 1260-1313).

After being strict about no caffeine for years, I have reintroduced even though it increases my trigger load. The side effects are unmistakable, as it causes spikes and crashes along with sustained changes in baseline, but I feel the benefits outweigh the impact. This is a highly personal evaluation, as for some this can never be ingested without significant impact[1] (Buchholz, Loc 1261, 1700-1710). An ongoing evaluation process is involved and if I reach a point where the balance of risk and reward has shifted, then I would react appropriately as I have done with many other foods and substances.

While I have reintroduced coffee and espresso, I remain strict around energy drinks. Espresso is preferable to other types of caffeine because it can be quickly consumed and followed by a glass of water, accelerating the return to hydration. Another strategy is to dilute espresso with water into an americano. Timing and trigger loads are essential considerations here because it causes minimal issues when consumed early in the day, but if I ingest it later in the day, the negative impact is significant.

Alcohol

As with all other dietary triggers previously discussed, this category certainly requires personalization. During the four-year period that I was strict, I eliminated alcohol completely. I have chosen to reintroduce alcohol even though I feel the impact on my system; some styles aggravate my migraine more than others. I manage this trigger, but it carries unique challenges.

The clear alcohols such as sake and vodka impact my migraine less than other styles such as beer, wine, and whiskey, as suggested in The 1-2-3 Program[1] (Buchholz, Loc 1393-1398). Alcohol is a perfect example in my case because it causes severe reactions, but in moderation it can be tolerated. Small amounts are more manageable when my overall trigger level is lower. Differences in diet, sleep, and exercise all change the impact of alcohol (or any other trigger), underscoring the importance of considering all variables in any test. When I enjoy alcohol, I am careful to balance that intake with periods of reduced trigger load. Not only do I try to minimize use before and after the period of intake, I also try to reduce exposure to other triggers simultaneously in order to compensate. Alcohol can cause a reaction based on any amount of consumption, but multiple days in a row certainly compounds the impact. This is true even in tests of small amounts, when consumed consistently there is clear impact to baseline and trigger sensitivity. Just as I have described with other triggers, I use alcohol as a reward. I remain strict in many scenarios, but I still explore when it is appropriate to be flexible.

One other related factor that has already been discussed is dehydration, as I certainly find the baseline impact to be minimized if I remain hydrated when I consume alcohol.

I enjoy this trigger using a long-term perspective. As with any of these examples, some may find alcohol easier to manage through complete elimination, but this is a personal decision. Overconsumption of alcohol can be catastrophic for migraine symptoms, as Dr. Buchholz suggests with his relation of migraine to an extreme hangover[1] (Buchholz, Loc 1396).

Reintroductions

While many of the above examples are items that I enjoy, a common thread involves foods that remain triggers. Many of these identified triggers have been added back into my diet successfully in moderation, such as chocolate, alcohol, caffeine, cheese, and bread. Others are completely unacceptable to me at this point, including bananas, citrus, certain nuts, processed meats, and additives (MSG[1], etc.). This is an ongoing exploration and as my perception of trigger impact changes I will continue to react when appropriate (Buchholz, Loc 1681-1745).

Medication

It is clear to me that as I move through this story, key lessons arise from my time on various medications. My personal experience with a variety of pharmaceuticals gives me a unique perspective on this category. My main objection is to the use of medication as a primary solution when the condition is mysterious. As I look back, the variety of drug categories we explored through trial and error delayed understanding of my issues because they added side effects to the equation.

Over the years, I consulted with multiple doctors and neurologists due to changing locations and insurance plans. I spent time in HMO plans and more flexible PPO plans. In the beginning, I was in an HMO and the first ten months of treatment involved drug testing with my primary care physician before he ever consulted with a neurologist. I was already deep in a pharmaceutical cloud by the time we took a more significant step and the neurologist then introduced the more extreme medications mentioned below. Cost must have been a factor in the decision by my initial doctor not to involve a neurologist earlier. If this amount of time had passed prior to the consultation with a neurologist in my father's case, there may have been more serious implications.

When I switched to a PPO and gained flexibility of provider, I was able to work with another neurologist who brought a different perspective. He referred me to The 1-2-3 Program[1] and offered unique solutions before helping move to a medication free approach at my direction. The tradeoff between cost and choice is a difficult one that must be weighed based on the unique variables involved.

I hesitate to consider specific medications out of concern that I may incorrectly bias others either for or against a specific treatment, or even treatment in general. Many of the principals that I suggest can be implemented without any change to current medical treatment. I also acknowledge that treatment options will hopefully evolve over time and so I do not intend to dismiss a future breakthrough based on personal results. This is certainly an area that must be approached with care in partnership with a competent doctor looking at the details of any situation. I am only going to revisit certain areas, with the goal of remaining focused on the importance of migraine management.

Migraine Medications

The list of pharmaceuticals I used in partnership with my doctors is long, there are many books[1] and resources previously published that could provide a more complete accounting of the various categories of pharmaceutical migraine treatment.

The general impact of this exploration is more important than the specific list of drugs. There were benefits at times, but the series of medications carried a variety of mental and physical side effects. It was often hard for me to distinguish the disease from the side effects and this must have also been the case for my doctors. I concede the potential benefits of these medications, but my concern is the fact that drug trial and error was the first treatment step, which complicated ongoing interpretation of symptoms. When no progress was made with one drug, we shifted to another and started all over again, rinse and repeat. The haze I entered under these pharmaceuticals took years to clear.

Anti-depressants. This was the first category of drugs that we tested when I presented with migraine. My recollection is that we tried at least three different anti-depressants before moving on to other categories, Amitriptyline is an example of this category. There were no noticeable benefits of these drugs, but there were two critical results from this treatment step.

The first result was the variety of side effects, including slowed reaction time and increased nausea. This reduced my ability to function during a time when I was already struggling with the basic activities of daily life.

The second result was much more concerning because this treatment undermined trust between me and my doctor. Anti-depressants are a legitimate treatment for migraine, but when I was initially prescribed this category it made me question the doctor's belief in my symptoms.

Prior to this treatment, I was already hesitant to report my symptoms because they were so mysterious. I only gave in and went to the doctor when I was desperate. This initial response of antidepressants left me with the inevitable feeling that he didn't believe my concerns. Even once I had confirmed that this category had prior success in treatment of migraine, I was still uncertain as to my primary doctor's true motivation in utilizing antidepressants first. To have the initial response create questions about trust was counterproductive.

Given the fact that the doctor didn't believe me, am I making up these symptoms? Is it all in my head and the doctor is treating me for delusional symptoms? Does the doctor believe that I am depressed? As I look back now, these questions seem like natural response to a treatment plan that indicates a lack of belief in the reported symptoms, but at the time they certainly made me insecure about my status.

As I have mentioned previously, antidepressants may be an effective treatment for some, but I do not feel that blindly throwing drugs at any problem is a solution. It is trial and error, so why start the trial this way?

Seizure Medication. This was where the mental cloud really took hold, as this category of drugs was much more powerful and carried a host of physical side effects that made my body feel (and sometimes act) like junk. Topamax and Depakote are the names that stand out in my memory, although there may have been others. Through this period, I was having significant difficulty functioning and my recollection is vague. As I look back, the sequencing is hard to recall in detail, which underscores the fog I was in at the time. I am confident this category was explored after anti-depressants and prior to lithium.

Lithium. This was the worst of anything that I was prescribed. Other uses for this drug include schizophrenia and a series of major psychological issues. The toll this took on my system was undeniable. An inability to function on a basic level, a complete lack of appetite, and a mental fog persisted even after we stopped this treatment.

In hindsight, the side effects were not worth the risk. I recall discussing this issue with my doctor prior to treatment, but I was so desperate for a solution that I did not take this as seriously as I should have at the time. I am confident that the side effects from this and other drugs were worse than any of my migraine symptoms.

Quick Fix Medication. This category includes everything from over the counter Excedrin Migraine to prescription short term solutions. Sumatriptan is one name that I recall, although there were a few others that we tried. I did not see any benefit in this category, but I had difficulty identifying the correct times to administer these 'proactive' drugs due to my ongoing discomfort. For those who have more definition in their spikes it may be more helpful. Even before reading The 1-2-3 Program[1], I had already moved past this treatment (Buchholz, Loc 730-1041).

Botox. During a period of a few years, we used Botox to freeze muscles through my head and neck. This took place in close partnership with my neurologist at the time and it was very early in the use of Botox for migraine treatment.

The doctor performed a series of Botox injections through my scalp on a quarterly basis, which helped break the migraine cycle. The injections were in strategic locations such as the bridge of my nose, along the hairline on my forehead, at the top of my neck, and in a few locations on my scalp under my hair.

This is the origin of the target areas for scalp massage and hair pulling discussed later, as I still try to achieve scalp relaxation even in the absence of Botox. These target points can be used effectively to penetrate my skull and relax my core.

Cannabis

There are a variety of myths around cannabis that stem from propaganda and nearly a century of prohibition. When I was in the darkest pits of my migraine, I was largely unable to eat, with all food tasting of ash. Many of the medications only contributed to that issue. The use of cannabis helps combat spikes and regain hunger for food. I reside in a state with a progressive approach to this alternative treatment, but local laws are important to consider before exploration.

One of the most interesting aspects of this exploration was the contrasting results from different strains of cannabis. There are many chemicals involved and different strains contain unique combinations. Some strains are very helpful, while others are counter-productive. The two main categories of strains are sativa and indica, but a variety of hybrids create a spectrum. While the strain is one variable, growing method also had an impact for me. Different sources should be tested since the same strains can vary significantly depending on cultivation conditions.

Some strains contain little or none of the most famous psychoactive cannabis ingredient, Delta-9 Tetrahydrocannabinol (THC), instead containing concentrations of other cannabinoids such as cannabidiol (CBD). These chemicals interact with our endocannabinoid system in ways that we do not yet fully understand, ongoing research is required. I found great benefit in the use of edible forms, especially high CBD tinctures and oils, which target the nausea directly and provide longer lasting results. Vaporization and smoking both have faster onset and dissipation, making these methods useful during extreme spikes. Topical creams are effective targeting specific muscles and joints.

Cannabis has interacted with my migraine struggle in positive ways, I am confident that it is an alternative to a variety of prescriptions and vices in society. Trial and error are required, which creates potential pitfalls if the wrong type is selected, just as with pharmaceuticals. This ongoing exploration of strains and the chemicals involved is a main benefit of ending prohibition, as doctors can finally apply modern scientific method to this broad category.

I theorized above that pharmaceuticals should not be a primary solution to migraine and there are similar risks to consider with cannabis. Given the scientific revolution we have experienced in the last century and the epidemic of addiction to pharmaceuticals, the classification process is clearly flawed. It is inconsistent to analyze drugs on two different spectrums (legal and illegal); we should consider them based on data rather than propaganda. Prohibition empowers black markets, escalates enforcement costs, and causes lost tax revenue, while increasing incarceration and not reducing addiction. We must end prohibition to unlock widespread research and education on all chemicals.

This research process is further along on cannabis in other countries and the initial results are encouraging for migraine patients. In 2017, a study[2] was presented to the European Academy of Neurology in Amsterdam demonstrating reductions in migraine pain from administration of combined THC and CBD. In the first phase, they explored dosages and found little benefit from small doses. Only when they administered higher doses was there a significant reduction in attacks. Phase two of the study involved administration of the successful dosages from phase one as compared to two conventional treatments, one for migraine and one for cluster headaches in different segments. These happened to be two of the drugs I was prescribed for a time, Amitriptyline and Verapamil. There was a significant reduction in migraine attacks during this phase of the study and the cannabis results slightly outperformed amitriptyline. There was also a similar reduction for cluster headache sufferers, although the positive results were isolated to patients who had experienced migraine since childhood. Side effects of the THC/CBD combination included drowsiness and difficulty concentrating. Ongoing research should explore varying chemical combinations of THC, CBD, and the other cannabinoids found in different strains of cannabis.

Further detail is available from many sources including Jack Herer's book "The Emperor Wears No Clothes" (1985), which discusses the history of cannabis.[3] Updated information on the evolving legal situation is available through NORML.org.[4] I look forward to the end of prohibition and the scientific renaissance on both positives and negatives of cannabis as it relates to migraine and many other areas.

Taosool

The Art of Standing on One Leg

I am not an exercise guru or a doctor, many of the techniques I utilize are highly customized and can be dangerous if applied incorrectly. This is not a comprehensive workout, as much of my exercise comes from exploration of the outdoors through hiking and skiing. As always, consult with your doctor as needed before beginning or changing any exercise routine.

Taosool is focused on mental and physical recovery, regeneration, relaxation, and flexibility. 'Standing on one leg' is both a physical action and a metaphor for managing symptoms while minimizing impact on daily goals. The progression should be careful, deliberate, and personal, allowing for anyone to start at a basic level and increase difficulty slowly. Proceed with caution when adapting any of these techniques to a different body, all variables must be considered in application.

Origins

The transition from a general focus on stability into what is now Taosool began on a slackline. We were camping near a river at high elevation when one member of the group set up a line between a tree and the trailer hitch on his truck. If you are not familiar, slacklining is essentially tightrope walking, but on flat webbing rather than round rope. Also, where traditional high wire acts are performed on a taught wire, with slacklining there is more flexibility in the line (as the name implies).

I attempted to walk the line and found it difficult, which is to be expected in the beginning. At one point while waiting for my turn on the line, I picked up one leg on solid ground to practice. I quickly realized that I was having difficulty standing on one leg in general rather than only on the line. Thus, I began to stand on one leg as much as possible. Slowly, but surely, my core strength improved and Taosool emerged.

As the migraine progressed, there were times where I didn't want to leave a dark room, but I needed to exercise my body. Taosool had already been a part of my routine, but at this point I began to expand use significantly. For many the gym is an effective place to work out, but I have always preferred the natural gym (outdoors) to any specific location. I now balance backcountry activity and Taosool as my main forms of exercise and recovery.

Early in the implementation of this strategy, I began to utilize it in my office cubicle. Often, I could be seen juggling various balls, stuffed animals, and objects while standing on one leg and talking on the phone. Many thanks to my nearby cubicle-mates, this juggling must have been distracting. More recently, this happens mostly in private although I have shared a few tips and tricks with friends and family.

Weight is only one measurement of success. My mental state, flexibility, and strength have all improved simultaneously with an improvement in fitness. At the point that I expanded use, my body weight was hovering just below 200 pounds, but now I am averaging around 150 pounds. There have been speed bumps in the road, discussed below under injuries, but the general trajectory has been positive since implementing this strategy. This trend continues through today and I experience ongoing improvement. When managing a difficult migraine spike, I use Taosool to target my discomfort regardless of surroundings.

Core Taosool

I allow my instincts to dictate the natural position rather than forcing my body to attain a certain pose at any given time. To accomplish this, I begin by standing straight with my feet a few inches apart. I raise one foot off the ground, often only an inch or two, but enough to shift my weight onto the other foot. I engage my core muscles and align myself upright over that single leg while maintaining an upright core posture.

Angling my legs, arms, and core in variations from this pose allows me to stretch and strengthen any muscle in my body with minimal impact. I use my hands in a simple and gentle motion, pushing or pulling energy in the necessary direction to provide balance. I open my mind and feel the presence of each muscle throughout my body, engaging them and striving for alignment.

When the anchor leg tires, I switch to the other and continue. Rather than repeating the exact motions, the switch is an extension of prior movement because my core is engaged the entire time. I return to similar base motions, but the sequence and length on each side varies. When I began, I could barely stand on one leg at all. With practice, each leg stand can be extended further.

The timing of anchor leg switch is grounded in my approach to hiking pace, where I try to maintain a pace that could continue indefinitely. Slow and steady wins the race. It is critical to push the boundaries of prior sessions or else there will be no progress, but overextension can lead to disaster. This is a very personal approach that must be customized appropriately, I work hard to let my body dictate what it needs.

When I discuss every muscle, I mean all the way up, not just through the legs. Much of my migraine tension is focused at the base of my skull where it connects to my upper vertebra, but this is a very difficult area to relax or massage. It is only through careful stretching and motion that certain areas can be released. I believe that engaging the core helps encourage a natural alignment throughout the body and target areas that would otherwise be unreachable.

The best part about this base motion is that it can be performed in nearly any location for zero cost. I enjoy doing this anywhere possible, such as in line at the supermarket, when brushing my teeth, and in the galley of an airplane. As the space allows, I expand from this base position into a variety of standing and sitting poses or stretches, with my body dictating focus.

Balance has improved significantly as I have developed this posture. The implications permeate my daily life, where I am more stable doing basic tasks such as climbing stairs. The positive impact spreads further, into more advanced activities such as skiing and hiking. Now that I am comfortable on one leg, many of the moves that would have seemed more difficult or exposed are much easier.

As I mentioned, this is not my main form of exercise because I am very active in my daily life, usually walking or hiking between two and ten miles in a day. Taosool is much more than just exercise, it improves my ability to breath, stretch, think, and recover. It has become a window to my core; a way to sense any unwanted tension in my body and help me understand my needs.

I relax into the stance, allowing the natural flow of energy to take over and dictate the target area. Quiet balance, neck stretching, and gentle hair pulling are most beneficial to migraine spike management. When my legs are sore and tired from a long hike or ski, I transition into a stretching focused sequence. My instincts command any movement from the core pose.

Basic Progression

There are a few basic Taosool motions that build the core stabilizing muscles throughout the body. I provide these as examples, but it is critical to underscore the fact that I remain flexible in these stances. Carefully attain improvement in each session, pushing the limits of core muscles by shifting the body in a variety of angles. Counter motion forces engagement of stabilizing muscles, sideways resistance can be added by shifting your weight.

Angel Step. A natural progression for me is often to bring the floating knee straight up in the air, forming as close to a natural ninety-degree angle at both my knee and hip. I try to straighten my back and neck, while also stretching and extending my anchor leg.

This name seems appropriate because the pose reminds me of a ski exercise from high school racing called the devil's chair, where we would sit against a wall with no chair. On multiple occasions, we closed practice with a competition to see who could last the longest. In Angel Step there are many similarities to this classic move, but I am suspended above the anchor leg with no wall for leverage. I attempt to achieve a similar ninety-degree angle at the knee and hip with my back straight and anchor leg straight or slightly bent. My arm position tends to float from vertical to horizontal as I use this opportunity to align my back, neck and shoulders while maintaining core posture.

Angel Side Step. The difficulty can be increased by opening or closing hips with the floating leg. Shifting between angel step and side step without moving core or lowering leg is very beneficial, this motion can be continuous from one side to the other with angel step as a midpoint.

There are potential similarities to a yoga tree pose when in angel side step stance depending on arm and leg position, but I see benefit in multiple leg positions from right to left and low to high along with arm positions at a variety of angles. Feel the comfortable position and push gently for posture improvement.

Knee Lifts. Stable on one leg with the floating leg just off the ground, lift knee forward into Angel Step and return to starting position. Repeat in sets, switching legs where appropriate. An advanced variation is to open or close hips and raise leg directly into angel side step.

Knee Bends. Bend the knee of the floating leg while keeping upper leg still, return to base position, repeat and switch legs as needed.

Knee Turns. Execute knee bend and hold. While maintaining stable core, turn at knee to swing floating foot out to one side, then turn back to the other side. Keep knee pointed down and isolate stretch in knee and hip. Repeat, switch anchor legs.

Straight Leg Lifts. With a straight floating leg, lifts can be performed forward, back, sideways, and diagonal. Lift only to comfortable height. Perform in sets, switching anchor legs. There is benefit in many angles here, including side to side variations once leg is extended.

Arm Circles. Extend arms out to side while on one leg, then swing arms in controlled circles. Vary circle size and direction, complete reps to comfort level. At least three sizes of circle should be used, but more are possible. Perform sets using each anchor leg, as target muscles change based on foundation.

Shoulder Turn. Maintain base position while spinning shoulders and upper body in both directions. Many arm positions are possible, but I prefer arms up in front with hands together and elbows out. I spin just that upper core and point the elbows forward/backward. This should also be performed on varying anchor legs to target core muscles.

Shoulder Roll. With arms in varying positions (high, low, front, back), roll shoulders repetitively in circles. Reverse direction and extend stretch in necessary directions.

Joint Sway and Turn. Shifting weight at different joints helps target specific areas. Either the upper or lower body can be turned, spread, or compacted to change center of gravity. This can be progressed into more advanced postures. As my position of comfort has expanded, I can now reach a more exaggerated position than I could initially; I am also comfortable branching off from that core position. It is essential to push the boundaries gently, rather than over extend.

With one leg in the air, there are multiple rotation points that must be explored throughout the core. Bend the anchor knee slightly and lift floating leg only a few inches off the ground, turn toes in and out while maintaining a straight leg and rotating at the hip. This simple move can effectively target many areas of the core. As comfort expands, this rotation can be performed at a variety of angles to target muscles further up in the core and upper body. Additional basic variations can be created through core rotation at top of either the anchor leg or floating leg.

I allow natural position to dictate my movement. My hands and arms flow in a gentle motion, pushing energy in any direction as needed to support balance. When I ground myself on one leg, I send energy through the bottom of my foot, extending roots into the ground.

Advanced Progression

Over time, these basic movements developed into more advanced maneuvers. I have provided examples below, but I stress the importance of customization and flexibility in these movements to target whatever areas of focus may be appropriate at that time.

Angel Step Circle. When in the core posture, raise knee straight in front. Open stance, rotating at hip without changing forward core posture. Swing leg in 'circle' back around to base position. Repeat in same direction for series of reps, then reverse direction and repeat set. Switch legs and repeat again. Only reach to natural limits of hip flexibility and balance.

Superperson. Swing floating leg behind and lean upper core forward. Extend arms, striving for ninety-degree angle at core hip joint in both directions. Working toward this stance is helpful in targeting various core areas. Feel core strengths and weaknesses and target them through the customized joint sway below.

Advanced Joint Sway. A great way to increase the difficulty of any posture is to add sway by turning and angling to increase complexity or target injuries. While stable on one leg, bend the anchor leg slightly and shift weight in and out on the anchor knee, which will angle the knee in and out, engaging stabilizing muscles. This must be done carefully, but when executed it can expand knee strength significantly. Keep core still, shifting weight in, out, forward and backward. Single leg squats are an advanced variation.

Rotation and stretching at each joint can be beneficial, including but not limited to hands, wrists, elbows, shoulders, spine/neck, core, hips, knees, ankles, and feet. Over time, this variety will significantly improve balance and longevity in stances.

This sway and rotation can be used at various joints, but neck stretching is the most beneficial for migraine. I use classic neck rolls to both sides, along with targeted directional stretching. Taosool enhances the connections that extend from the neck through the core. I often use the hair pull strategy (below) to anchor my head and neck in a certain position, then I can apply internal pressure to spread my spine from my skull effectively.

Ski Skating. For cardio work, I target my skiing focus, which is on my mind all times of year. Creativity should be applied in the customization of any strategy toward personal goals and interests. You must know your limits. If you overextend there could be serious consequences so be very careful about traction and stance. Start by setting two imaginary lines outside shoulder width. Then stand on one leg at that boundary and jump to the other leg, landing at the opposite target and regaining balance on one leg. Repeat, varying pace and width.

As regaining balance when jumping from leg to leg becomes standard, the motion can be extended into more advanced maneuvers by landing and swinging the floating leg in front or behind the anchor leg. Periods of increased pace are best combined with targeted relaxed poses; this increases heart rate through the session and enhances enjoyment.

Taosool Principals

The physical action of standing on one leg is only the beginning, as the basic methods of Taosool can be used to combat migraine in a variety of situations. Creativity is key, as I customize my approach to the challenge at hand.

Breathing. I have exercise induced asthma that has required management all my life and breathing is critical in controlling pace. When I am not focused on my breathing, I use my nose or mouth, but not both. I naturally breathe more through my nose when at rest and mostly through my mouth when exercising. My focus and performance in all areas is improved when I balance this breathing, in through the nose and out through the mouth. I use breathing to create mental and physical peace during any activity.

In through the nose, out through the mouth. Repeat. Adjust pace.

Hair Pull and Self Massage. I massage my head and body in various areas, specifically around the eye sockets, near the temples, throughout the scalp, and around the upper neck. I allow my discomfort to dictate the areas of focus. By adding this to a variety of stances in Taosool, I relax areas that would otherwise be unreachable.

General manipulation of the skin is also beneficial. A common area of focus for this strategy is the bridge of my nose through my eyebrows, but a gentle pinch or pull encourages muscle relaxation in many areas. Manual shifting and stretching of my ears targets the side of the scalp.

Hair pulling is an extension of the muscle targeting in each pose and the connection runs all the way through my core. A gentle pull separates my scalp from my skull and helps relax the core muscles. I reiterate the gentle nature of this move, as I am not pulling my hair to create pain. The power of this move is to stretch not hurt. By grasping small clumps of hair, one or two at a time, I separate my scalp from my skull in different directions: up, down, side to side, and everything in between. In addition to pulling the scalp away from the skull, shifting the scalp along the skull creates a satisfying sensation. Hair pull is an effective technique for me when I am in the worst spikes.

This hair pull can be used when sitting at a desk or any other location, but I will provide an example of an effective progression. With both feet on the ground, shoulder width apart, lean forward with legs straight but knees unlocked. Relax spine, reach for toes without overextending, breathe deeply and settle into stretch. Reach back with both hands and gently pull hair or skin at back of neck. Focus on the muscle connection from scalp through neck into core. Target sore areas, relax and breathe while continuing to massage scalp and gently pull hair in different directions.

While this example reflects use of hair pull in a standard forward stretch, it is very useful in any posture. The essential component is a counterweight approach in order to access the core structure. When on either leg, different muscles can be engaged by pulling on the same side of the head as the anchor leg versus the opposite. It is essential to feel the connections running throughout the body.

Meditation and Sensory Deprivation. I have never been formally trained in meditation, but I have a natural understanding of basic principles that help me manage my mental state. Rather than resort to traditional methods I follow my instincts and they serve me well. It is my belief that this true core is different for everyone, which makes it even more critical to take a personal approach.

Meditation is very beneficial in obtaining the mental power necessary to conquer chronic migraine. As I developed my abilities, I learned to expand my core focus under varying conditions, such as when I am riding out a significant migraine spike in an uncomfortable location. These sessions have a positive impact on both the body and the mind that is highly personalized.

Sensory deprivation is helpful to encourage meditation, I have experimented with use of a float tank to achieve this state. The pod is large enough to lay down in ten inches of salt water, with a manual lid and a private room including shower. Sounds and lights can remain on throughout the session, but I prefer total darkness and silence. This environment brings out a higher level of focus with less concentration than is required in a more chaotic location. I had difficulty settling in during the initial sessions, but it is easier with practice. As I improved my ability to detach in the tank, it became much easier to meditate outside the tank.

The initial posture is on my back with my feet shoulder width apart and my hands floating palms down a comfortable distance from my sides. As I settle in, the water supports my body into a flat position, and I work to relax each resistant area. These target areas present at various times during the session. Sometimes a stretch of the area is effective, but angling other parts of the body in interesting ways can target a variety of locations.

Shoulder position is essential. I usually begin hunched over, but by rolling my shoulders back and shifting them in all directions I achieve a satisfying stretch. I rotate and stretch my shoulders while maintaining the rest of my core steady, although it requires an engaged core to remain still in the water as you begin to move extremities. As my upper body relaxes, the base position shifts and I enter a more natural posture within the water. I progress through my entire body, continuing this alignment through any problem areas.

Slow and deliberate motions help maintain suspension in the water. Just like when upright in Taosool, the core is essential in this situation, so I begin in a base position and allow my body to dictate progression. I maintain my core horizontally in line with the top plane of the water, simultaneously engaging and relaxing every muscle in my body, searching for alignment.

Rotating my arms and legs at each joint can be effective, just like the joint sway or twist above when on one leg. Since this action is performed while suspended in salt water, it is key to keep your eyes and face protected. Once salt contamination occurs, the session is effectively over. I also suggest wax earplugs, which are much more comfortable than other alternatives and will keep salt water out.

As my strategy expanded, I experimented with the timing of tank use. For instance, after a plane ride there is significant relaxation benefit. In one case after a long flight, I slept in the pod and woke up incredibly refreshed.

When I am exhausted and in need of time to unwind, it is much easier to engage in the session. Conversely, if I am highly energetic it is more difficult to settle into the tank. Floating is worthwhile in either scenario, although the impact differs. The sessions where I begin more relaxed are more likely to expand consciousness, but the basic relaxation that can be achieved during a hectic session is also very helpful. Completing the full session is preferable because the return of light is a pleasant welcome back to reality, like a sunrise waking my body from slumber.

Sensory deprivation is an interesting example of how reality changes in darkness. Theoretical physics is outside the scope of this discussion, but my perception of time slows to a crawl during these sessions. This allows for highly complex thoughts to take place in an efficient manner. As the light returns, I experience an acceleration of time. The final five minutes of light flies by, even when time seemed to be moving very slowly in the darkness.

This state is helpful in a variety of locations and situations in order to overcome migraine spikes. Darkness and silence can be replicated, but they are not required. One strategy here is to find an isolated dark room for meditation. When working in an office building, a vacant conference room away from busy areas was useful. This meditation was effective sitting or lying down, but Taosool can increase the versatility of these sessions by pairing core exercise with meditation.

While I still enjoy floating and feel major benefits, Taosool has become my main access point to this meditative release. The tank is helpful in training, but this same meditation can be executed in any location when I encounter a significant migraine spike.

Brain Relaxation. One of the most important muscles in this process in the brain, which is just as critical to release as any other area. The inside of the skull is very difficult to reach, but with care it can be targeted just like any other core muscle. I have the most success targeting this area through Taosool due to the combination of mental and physical exercise. Mental exercise can be performed anywhere, whether standing on one leg, lying in a sensory deprivation tank, or standing on a street corner. To accomplish this, I expand my focus to include everything around me.

> Reach out with the mind, focus on everything and nothing.
>
> Expand consciousness and sink into the environment.
>
> Align posture with universe.

Finding this mental center leads to a relaxation of the mind. Balance improves as the level of comfort in the stance increases, which is why

Taosool is not ridged and instead is more flexible. This expanded focus encourages energy to flow freely; I aim to achieve a balancing of energy.

Often, this mental exercise will reveal an issue of importance. I theorize that when the mind settles, it allows the subconscious an opportunity to dictate focus, accessing deep instincts that are otherwise inaccessible. The constant noise of our fast-paced technological society makes it even more essential for everyone to engage and release this muscle. Tapping into both the internal and external neural network using meditation can help expand consciousness.

Injury recovery. I have a long list of injuries and the need to rehab was a driving motivation in the initial exploration of Taosool. It is critical to emphasize that I have no expectation of my techniques eliminating injury, but I am confident they have aided in my ability to function through migraine, manage pain, and relax areas that would otherwise be unreachable.

This approach to stabilizing muscles dates back prior to my migraine issues, as I have recovered from a variety of injuries over the years. My lower leg issues began with a dislocated kneecap which tore the meniscus and sprained my ACL, leading to scar tissue that was cleaned out in a relatively minor procedure. I have been lucky not to cause major structural damage, but to avoid this moving forward I work to strengthen the knee muscles. Core strength from head to toe has made my knees stronger than ever. This did not happen overnight; patience and discipline have been essential.

A few years ago, I tore my Achilles tendon when skiing with friends. While I mostly ski in powder and trees, that day we were going top speed down a groomer in early season. As we came around a corner and pumped over a roller, I caught an edge and went down hard. The tip of my ski dug into the snow during the tumble and twisted my lower leg beyond normal range of motion.

A good Samaritan first responder stopped and helped with an initial evaluation. I was able to put weight on it, even though I was certainly in pain, so we decided to avoid ski patrol and allow me to work my way down the mountain. This was only the second run of the day and we were still just warming up for the season, so I encouraged my friends to continue skiing while I skied the "easiest way" back to the base.

At this resort it was not just a matter of skiing down, there were a variety of slopes I had to navigate in order to return. This distance was mostly covered on my one remaining good leg, with the injured leg dangling. Anything other than vertical pressure was extremely painful. Fairly certain I had injured my Achilles, I recalled Greek mythology as I worked my way down to the base, where I camped out for the day watching football and self-medicating while my friends enjoyed the snow. I would have remained in the ski boot for much longer if it were not for the help of one specific waitress, who literally pulled my ski boot off in the restaurant as I yelled out in pain.

While I knew immediately that I had injured myself, I did not feel it was necessary to see a doctor because I trusted my instincts. After a month of rest, I began self-directed rehab, which included Taosool and continuing to ski through most of the season. It appears the ski boot acted like an early walking boot, I felt more stable on skis than off and had a decent season on a partially torn Achilles.

When I finally went to the doctor four months later at the urging of my masseuse, he confirmed that I had self-diagnosed correctly, but I had not given myself enough rest. After time in a boot and on a scooter, I engaged in physical therapy to work my leg back into shape. I was still able to stand on the other leg when I was in the walking boot, although at the instruction of my doctor I put minimal intentional strain on the Achilles itself until we started rehab.

Even after this period of atrophy in the boot, my stabilizing structure was intact, and I was able to progress quickly through many of the activities at physical therapy. While there were multiple exercises we performed, one stands out in my memory. The therapist laid out a rope ladder and explained how to jump through, but with very little coaching I was able to stand on one leg and jump in a variety of patterns. It was clear from her reaction that this was well beyond expectations given my ability to perform other basic motions with my lower leg. Because of the stabilizing structure I was able to push the limits. Injuries can happen to anyone and Taosool will not prevent injury, but it has assisted in my preparation and recovery.

Customization. This approach is very personal, as it is customized to my needs. In my case, I wanted to be able to ski and hike at an expert level regardless of bad knees. Many of the stances are very focused on the muscles associated with those actions. Over time, other goals have emerged including migraine management and an Achilles tear; I have adapted these techniques around my evolving personal needs.

Creativity is essential, although care is required to avoid injury. I am sure ongoing disclaimer is appropriate, DO NOT start any exercise routine without consulting your doctor!

As I document my approach, I have intentionally avoided the use of strict poses in order to encourage imagination rather than imitation. Once you are comfortable on one leg, the key is to allow your instincts to dictate focus.

It occurs to me that some may not be able to execute these actions in their described form due to a difference in body function. I encourage participation in mental and physical exercise by anyone regardless of ability and these principals can be applied in a variety of ways. I have two functioning legs and a healthy core, but some do not. Personalized exploration of body and mind is the power of Taosool, even though there may be fundamental differences in application.

Taosool has significant benefits in my daily migraine management, but it also helps improve my ability to function in other ways. This account is focused on the migraine applications, but the potential uses for these basic techniques are vast and flexible.

Conclusion

The role of pharmaceuticals as the initial step in migraine treatment must be reevaluated by the medical community. My road was complicated due to a variety of prescription medications and their side effects, many of which were worse than the migraine symptoms. We continue to see breakthroughs that combat major concerns so we must embrace a scientific perspective on all chemicals while simultaneously reducing abuse of any category.

I control my migraine symptoms mainly through diet, exercise, and meditation. My instincts lead the way when eating, standing on one leg, exploring backcountry situations, or evaluating other decisions encountered through life. I have conditioned myself to feel the pain and work through it rather than turning to an external solution. It is only through trial and error that I have identified triggers and made progress managing them.

This is intended as my personal migraine case study, a contribution to the record that seems required due to my unique perspective and strategies. I am confident that my ability to function is enhanced through the techniques discussed above. Rather than delay access to these thoughts in order to include other sources and add detail, I am self-publishing to spark the conversation.

I make no claims of perfection. One of the core tenants of American society is the free and open ability to question ideas without fear of implications. I look forward to a spirited debate on these topics and I hope that scientific exploration will continue to progress into a new era.

Acknowledgement

At one point, a neurologist referred me to a book called "Heal your Headache: The 1-2-3 Program for Taking Charge of your Pain", by Dr. David Buchholz (2002). I used the food list as the base for my elimination diet, although I took it to an extreme and eliminated many other items not on that list through my personal testing.

I thank Dr. Buchholz for his work, much of his language is a part of my migraine dialect and I have shared his book with countless friends, family, and strangers. I do not intend to infringe on the ideas he presented, but rather to expand the discussion through documentation of my case.

When necessary, the title has been abbreviated and cited to maintain flow of text. Dr Buchholz was comprehensive so it should be considered a prerequisite for anyone experiencing migraine. In editing, I have sourced and cross-referenced comprehensively with Kindle locations.

References

1) Buchholz, D. (2002). *Heal Your Headache: The 1-2-3 Program for Taking Charge of your Pain.* Workman Publishing. New York.

2) Congress of the European Academy of Neurology. (June 24, 2017). *Cannabinoids suitable for migraine prevention.* https://www.ean.org/amsterdam2017/fileadmin/user_upload/E-EAN_2017_-_Cannabinoids_in_migraine_-_FINAL.pdf. Accessed 3/26/2019.

3) Herer, Jack. (1985). *The Emperor Wears No Clothes.* Ah Ha Pub. Van Nuys, CA.

4) NORML. (2019). NORML.ORG. Accessed 3/26/2019.

Made in United States
Troutdale, OR
11/03/2026

56845103R00080